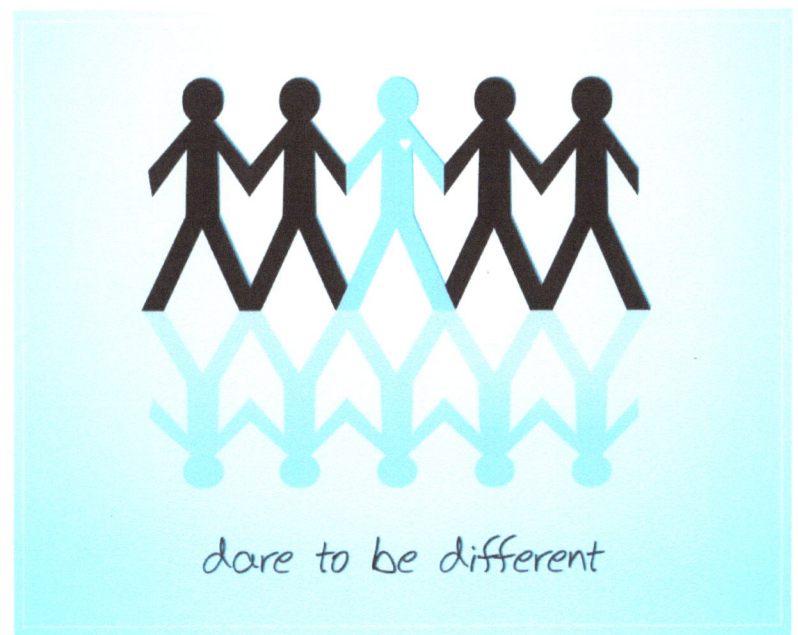

dare to be different

By

Rhiannon M Powell
Mental Health Advocate (Retired)

Acknowledgements
My sincere thanks to Mr John Boardman, Mr Paul Cowans , Dr David Ellis, Ms Ann Hardman, Mr Roger Moss, Dr Seshagiri Rao Nimmagadda, Ms Sandie Powell, Mr Peter Slater, and Mr S. Mohammed without whom this publication would never have happened.

CONTENTS

CULTURAL AND RELIGIOUS ISSUES AND MENTAL HEALTH

INTRODUCTION

This guidance (and it is by no means comprehensive) looks at some of the ways in which the needs of people, whatever their cultural or religious background, can be met during a hospital stay.

The aim is to increase awareness of differing beliefs, worship, diets, rites, birth, marriage and death helping all to *"respond appropriately and with sensitivity."*

There are several common factors which cause mental distress in all communities such as:

- difficulties in preserving identify and culture

- disintegration of historical and cultural values

- racism (including being made to feel guilty about receiving the health care to which they are entitled.)

- separation from family and loved ones

- inadequate housing

- language barriers. (If possible a professional interpreter should be employed rather than a family member who may lack objectivity.)

A racist incident is any incident which is perceived to be racist by the victim or any other person. This means if anyone thinks it is a racist incident, then it is.

Roots

The Anglican churches are a worldwide group of churches which recognise as their head (or primate) the Archbishop of Canterbury. The Church of England is the established or state church in England and part of this worldwide Anglican Communion, as is the Church in Wales.

Henry VIII started the process of creating the Church of England after his split with the Pope in the 1530s. Henry was anxious to ensure a male heir after his first wife, Catherine of Aragon, had borne him only a daughter. He wanted his marriage annulled in order to remarry. In 1534 after several attempts to persuade the Pope to grant an annulment, Henry passed the Act of Succession and then the Act of Supremacy. These recognised that the King was *"the only supreme head of the Church of England called Anglicana Ecclesia."* Henry adopted the title given to him by the Pope in 1521, that of Defender of the Faith. Today the Queen is the Supreme Governor of the church (theologically Jesus Christ is the head). On accession, the Prince of Wales wishes to become "Defender of the Faiths."

Though there is clear evidence of a Christian presence in Wales during the Roman occupation, the evangelisation of the people of Wales can be traced back to St David in the fifth and sixth centuries. Over time the fourth ancient dioceses of the Welsh church became part of the province of Canterbury. After a lengthy campaign in the late 19th and early 20th centuries, the Welsh dioceses of the Church of England were disestablished by Parliament in 1920 and the Church in Wales was formed. Like all Anglican churches, it recognises the primacy of the Archbishop of Canterbury who does not have any formal authority in Wales. This means that, unlike England, Wales no longer has a state church.

Beliefs

Broadly the beliefs of the Anglican Church are:

- that the Bible contains the core of all Christian faith and thought;

- a loyalty to a way of worship and life as set out in the Book of Common Prayer;

- celebration of the sacraments ordained by Jesus;

Festivals/Days of Observance

The main festivals are:

- Christmas marks the birth of Jesus, the son of God.

- Epiphany celebrates the visit of the Wise Men from the East to see the baby Jesus.

- Lent is the period of forty days which comes before Easter in the Christian calendar, traditionally a time of fasting and reflection. It is preceded by Shrove Tuesday (Christians seek forgiveness for their sins and prepare for Lent) and begins with Ash Wednesday.

- Holy Week is the week leading up to Easter, beginning on Palm Sunday (the entry of Jesus into Jerusalem), including Maundy Thursday and ending on Holy Saturday.

- Easter is the most important Christian festival. It celebrates Jesus Christ's resurrection from the dead, three days after he was crucified.

- Pentecost/Whitsun – this commemorates when the followers of Jesus received the Holy Spirit.

Essential Information

Baptism marks becoming a member of the local and worldwide Christian family. When a child is baptised, the parents/guardians make public declarations, on behalf of the child, that you believe in God and that the child will be brought up to follow Jesus. The Church of England emphasises that marriage should always be undertaken as a *'solemn, public and life-long covenant between a man and a woman.'*

When a Christian dies, a funeral is held to grieve for the person and give thanks for their life. The funeral service of the Church of England can be very short and quiet with only a few members of the family present or an occasion of great solemnity with music, hymns and a packed church.

The Church of England combines strong opposition to abortion with a recognition that there can be strictly limited conditions under which it may be morally preferable to any available alternative. The Church of England does not regard contraception as a sin or a contravention of God's purpose.

Euthanasia, as precisely defined, is not compatible with the Christian faith and the Church distinguishes between euthanasia and withholding, withdrawing, declining or terminating excessive medical treatment and intervention, all of which enable a person to die with dignity. When a person is in a permanent vegetative state, to sustain him or her with artificial nutrition and hydration may be seen as constituting medical intervention.

ATHEISM/HUMANISM

Beliefs

Atheism, broadly speaking, is the absence of belief in deities or gods. Individuals live as if there are no gods and explain natural phenomena without resorting to the divine. The existence of gods is not denied but they believe that gods neither provide purpose to life, nor influence their everyday life.

Humanism is an approach to life based on humanity and reason. Humanists recognise that moral values are properly founded on human nature and experience alone. Decisions are based on the available evidence and an assessment of the outcomes of these actions, not on any dogma or sacred text. Humanists believe that we should all try to live full and happy lives and that this includes helping other people to do the same.

Festivals/Days of Observance

Humanists like to celebrate, but prefer to do so in non-religious ceremonies, where they will not find themselves saying things they do not believe.

- In February, Imbolc (also called Oimelc and Candlemas) celebrates the awakening of the land and the growing power of the sun.

- Spring Equinox (21st March) – night and day stand equal.

- Beltane (1st May) – Pagans celebrate with maypole dances symbolising the mystery of the sacred marriage of goddess and god.

- Midsummer (21st June) – the festival of summer solstice. It is a time of plenty.

- Lughnasadh (1st August) – the time of the corn harvest when Pagans give thanks and reap those things they have sown.

- Autumn Equinox (21st August) – day and night stand equal.

- Samhain (31st October) – the festival of the dead when Pagans remember those who have gone before and acknowledge the mystery of death. Pagans celebrate death as a part of life.

- Yule (21st December) – the winter solstice.

Essential Information

Humanists may choose to have a baby naming ceremony or welcoming ceremony – with or without an Humanist celebrant. The parents sometimes choose guardians or mentors to act as supporting adults who will take a special interest in the child. The ceremony can take place anywhere, but is often held at home.

Humanist weddings/civil partnerships are very likely to take place in a Registry Office (the legal part of getting married) but many people may want to choose their own words of commitment to each other. They can ask friends or family to officiate at the wedding, or use an experienced celebrant. Some religions will not conduct weddings for divorced couples or for couples of different faiths, or ceremonies for gay couples, but Humanist ceremonies are available to everyone.

Humanists accept death as natural and inevitable, and often plan their own funerals before they die. There is no suggestion that the person has gone on to another life. They do not pray, though humanist funerals will often include a brief silence when people can reflect or pray if they want to.

Morally many humanists may believe that they have a responsibility to allow their organs to be used if, by donating organs after their death, they can help someone else. Donating an organ as a live donor, for example a kidney, is also within their code and the individual's own decision.

BAHA'I

Roots

Sayyid Ali Muhammad was born in Shiraz, Iran (then Persia) in 1819. He believed he was the messenger of God and called himself the Báb meaning *'gate'*. Part of his mission was to prepare the way for the coming of a greater messenger. His new religious movement culminated in a fierce persecution of its adherents as Islamic heretics and in 1850 he was executed. Mirza Husayn Ali Nuri (1817-1892), from Tehran, a follower of the Báb, took the name Bahá'u'lláh, which means *'The glory of God'*, and went on to found the Bahá'í faith. Bahá'u'lláh wrote many letters and key works in his lifetime and these are all regarded as part of Bahá'í scriptures.

Beliefs

The Bahá'í teachings maintain that the purpose of life in this world is to show to the greatest extent possible such spiritual qualities as love, justice, patience, compassion, wisdom, purity and trustworthiness.

Festivals/Days of Observance

The nine Bahá'í holy days commemorate events in the life of the Bab and Bahá'u'lláh. This includes the Bahá'í New Year, which falls on 21st March (the first day of Spring). This is a holiday. The Bahá'í calendar has nineteen months of nineteen days.

- Feast of the Ascension of Bahá'u'lláh - This commemorates the anniversary of the death of Bahá'u'lláh (29th May).

- Feast of the Birth of the Báb – To celebrate the birth of Báb (20th October).

- Feast of the Declaration of the Báb - This holy day celebrates the Báb's announcement of his mission. (22-23 May, from 2 hours after sunset on the 22nd).

- Feast of the Martyrdom of the Báb - This commemorates the events surrounding the death of the Báb in 1850. (9th July).

- Naw-Rúz - Literally *'new day'* is the Bahá'í new year festival. (21st March).

- Ridván - This Festival marks Bahá'u'lláh's time in the garden of Ridván and his announcement that he was the prophet promised by the Báb. (Sunset 21 April to sunset 2 May).

Essential Information

Bahá'ís believe that each human being has an immortal soul. The family is the bedrock of the individual's spiritual development and the foundation for society's stability. Family planning is left to personal conscience but sterilisation of either sex is unacceptable. Divorce is strongly discouraged but, if there are irreconcilable differences and a strong aversion between the partners, then divorce is permitted after a year, during which time efforts should be made for reconciliation. Bahá'ís may not be cremated or embalmed and should not be buried more than an hour's journey from the place of death. The family (or the local assembly of the Bahá'ís) will arrange the funeral. They may leave their bodies to scientific research or donate organs, if they wish.

Daily prayer and reflection on the sacred writings is obligatory. Bahá'ís believe strongly in the power of prayer in healing.

Diet

Bahá'ís is free of rituals and they do not have to eat any special kind of food nor wear special clothing. Some Bahá'ís may be vegetarian by choice. Generally they do not use habit-forming drugs and do not drink alcohol. Smoking is discouraged but not prohibited.

BAPTIST

Roots

The modern Baptist movement was born in the 16th century and is now a worldwide denomination with millions of believers worshipping in Baptist congregations. In 1612 the first Baptist church met in Spitalfields, London. Thomas Helwys, a founder of the Baptist denomination, published *'A Short declaration of the mystery of iniquity'*, calling for religious liberty. In the 17th century Baptists refused to conform and be members of the Church of England, arguing that Christ, and not the King (or Queen) was head of the church. They were persecuted for their beliefs.

Beliefs

Baptists do not have one distinctive Baptist belief. It is a combination of various beliefs, which make Baptists distinctive. Common beliefs for Baptists are the Lordship of Christ, the authority of the Bible, Baptism for believers, a believers' Church, the priesthood of all believers, church members and church meeting, interdependence, sharing the faith and religious freedom. In the Baptist movement everyone is equal. There is no hierarchy of bishops or priests.

There are five key values that guide the life of a Baptist:

- A Prophetic Community

- An Inclusive Community

- A Sacrificial Community

- A Missionary Community

- A Worshipping Community Festivals/Days of Observance.

Essential Information

To be baptised is a way of receiving God's blessing and of expressing commitment to lives as disciples of Christ. A baptism in a Baptist church is nearly always by full immersion. Many Baptist churches have baptismal pools at the front of the church that are often hidden under the floor, with steps going down into it.

BUDDHIST

Roots

Siddhartha Gautama (The Buddha) who was born around the year 580 BC, was led from the pain of suffering and rebirth towards the path of Enlightenment and became known as the Buddha or *'awakened one'*.

Beliefs

Buddhism is a tradition that focuses on personal spiritual development. Buddhists strive for a deep insight into the true nature of life and do not worship gods or deities. The basic teachings and concepts in Buddhism are:

- Karma - Actions have consequences; so our lives are conditioned by our past actions.

- Rebirth - Consciousness continues after death, and finds expression in a future life.

- Liberation from karma - By following the Buddha's path one escapes the cycle of craving and suffering.

The Four Noble Truths, the essentials of Buddhism are:

- Enlightenment - The highest goal of life is to reach Enlightenment; a state of being that goes beyond suffering.

- Dharma - The teachings and hence the way to Nirvana.

- The core of Buddhist teaching - At the heart of the Buddha's teaching lie The Four Noble Truths and The Eightfold Path which lead the Buddhist towards the path of Enlightenment.

- Facing the truth - The Buddha taught that the human tendency is to avoid the difficult truths of life and this in turn leads to suffering. By enabling the mind to be at peace through meditation a human being can confront reality and overcome hatred and craving.

Most Buddhists worship at home, where there will be a shrine including a statue of the Buddha, candles and an incense burner. Buddhists do not worship the statue, but they may bow to it as an expression of respect and gratitude, and they use it as a reminder of the virtues they need to develop to reach enlightenment.

Festivals/Days of Observance

Among the major celebrations are:

- Buddhist New Year - This depends on the country of origin or ethnic background of the people.

- Pavinirvana - marks the final passing away of the Buddha.

- Vaisakha Puja/Wesak - celebrates the birthday, enlightenment and death of Buddha.

- Dhammacakka/Asalha - Commemorates Buddha's first sermon of Benares in India.

- Bodhi Day - Some Buddhists celebrate Buddha's attainment of enlightenment (Nirvana).

Essential Information

There are no specific Buddhist birth rites but in some Buddhist countries boys aged between eight and 20 enter a monastery for a short time and experience life as a novice monk. The form a Buddhist wedding ceremony takes varies according to the particular tradition and the individual wishes of the couple. In Britain, couples may invite a monk to chant at the end of a secular ceremony, or they may have a ceremony with more of a Buddhist focus, led by a monk. Buddhist funeral rites differ widely according to the region, but central to most ceremonies is the idea that death is inevitable and grieving, though understandable, is without purpose. In Britain, the funeral can reflect any of these variations dependent on the wishes and tradition of the deceased.

There are no objections to blood transfusions or transplants. Most Buddhists believe that sickness is the result of their previous lives. The size of the family is dictated by destiny and, as far as family planning is concerned, this should not be interfered with. If used, then it should be a method which safeguards the normal development of the baby. Buddhist tradition condemns abortion. Helping people is fundamental to Buddhists and so the patient will respect the doctor, nurses and other professionals for helping him/her.

Diet

Eating fish and meat is allowed in Buddhism, though vegetarianism is encouraged. Buddhists eat merely to sustain the physical body and without greed, without craving for any kind of food, and without direct involvement in the killing of any animal.

CATHOLIC

Roots

The Roman Catholic Church can trace its history back almost 2000 years. The apostles of Jesus Christ formed the beginnings of the Christian Church. They helped spread the Gospel and provided structure for the early Church. It is hard to differentiate the beginnings of the Roman Catholic Church from that of the early Christian church. The apostle, Peter, also known as Simon, was of central importance and the Church was organized and presided over by him. Catholics believe that the Pope, based in Rome, is the successor to Saint Peter.

Catholics suffered a long period of persecution following Henry VIII's break with the Pope in the 1530s. By the start of the nineteenth century, *'anti-popery'* prejudices started to die away and full civic rights were restored in 1829.

Beliefs

Catholics endeavour to be true disciples of Jesus following his example and his teachings. They seek forgiveness of their sins. They believe that Jesus has provided seven Sacraments which give Grace from God to the believer.

Unless a Catholic dies in unrepented mortal sin, which is absolved in the Sacrament of Penance or Reconciliation (Confession), it is believed that person has God's promise of inheriting eternal life. Before entering heaven, some undergo a purification, known as Purgatory.

Catholic social teaching emphasizes love, forgiveness, charity towards others, especially those most in need, and respect for the sanctity of life.

Festivals/Days of Observance

In addition to the days celebrated by the Anglican Group of Churches, the Catholic Church also celebrates Holy days of Obligations for England and Wales (when Catholics are expected to attend Holy Mass, if possible). These are:

- Every Sunday

- Birth of the Lord (25 December)

- St Peter & St Paul (29 June)

- Assumption of the Blessed Virgin Mary (15 August)

- All Saints (1 November).

The following celebrations have been transferred to the nearest Sunday:

- Epiphany of the Lord

- Ascension of the Lord

- Body and Blood of the Lord

Essential Information

Baptism is the sacrament which makes one a member of the Church. The person being baptised is washed with holy water. This signifies the washing away of original sin and being reborn to a new life in Christ.

The Church promotes the value of virginity before marriage and of constancy. Divorce is immoral and introduces disorder into the family and into society. Innocent victims of civil divorce, however, are not guilty. Birth control except by natural methods is against Catholic belief as are reproductive technologies that substitute for the marriage act.

Catholics believe in life after death, that good people will rise again on the last day and live forever as Christ has done. At death, the body and soul are separated, *'the human body decays and the soul goes to meet God, while waiting its reunion with its glorified body.'*

The Catholic Church opposes activities that it believes destroy or devalue divinely created life, including euthanasia, eugenics and abortion.

The Catholic Church teaches that homosexual people *'must be accepted with respect, compassion, and sensitivity'* and is not considered sinful or evil in itself. Homosexual orientation that leads to sexual activity is found by the church to be disordered.

Diet

The practice of not eating meat on a Friday was discontinued many years ago. Nevertheless some Catholics do prefer to eat fish on Fridays (and always on Good Friday).

CHINESE

Roots

The Chinese have a rich and very varied tradition with an often complex system of magical belief and practice. China is the home to one of the world's oldest and most complex civilisations covering a history of over 5,000 years. In terms of numbers, however, the pre-eminent ethnic group is the Han Chinese.

Beliefs

See under Buddhism and Taoism Confucianism is based on the teachings and writings of the philosopher Confucius. It is an ethical belief system rather than a religion, and is based upon the concept of relationships. In Confucianism every relationship has the dual aspect of responsibility and obligation. Therefore the relationship between mother and child, husband and wife, brother and sister all have responsibilities and obligations. However, Confucianism goes beyond the family, and incorporates the relationship of individuals with the state, subject and ruler, bureaucrat and civilian. If these responsibilities and obligations are observed, then society will be a just and harmonious one.

Festivals/Days of Observance

The Chinese celebrate major festivals such as Christmas, New Year and Easter. Even though most Chinese, especially those who do not have a Christian faith, do not attach religious significance to these festivals, they all see them as an opportunity for fun, a break from their work routine, a time for family reunion, as well as an opportunity for good business.

Among the numerous Chinese festivals with traditions and rituals observed are:

- Qing Ming, Chong Yang (Double Nine Festival)

- Zuo Dong (Winter)

- Yu Lan Festival (Chinese Halloween)

- Chinese (or Lunar) New Year

- Teng Chieh – This marks the first full moon of the year. Chinese people celebrate the Lantern festival on this day.

- Ch'ing Ming – around the 5th April, the Chinese visit their family tombs. Sweeping and tidying takes place and offerings of food and wine are made to the spirits of the dead.

- Dragon Boat Festival (also known as Duan Wu Festival) – a festival held in honour of China's great poet Ch'u Yuan.

- Mid-Autumn Festival (also known as Moon Cake Festival).

The mother may be unwilling to go and have a bath during the first few days after birth as traditionally she would rest at this time. About a month after birth, the baby's head is shaved.

Funerals and mourning vary widely in Chinese tradition. On the death of an infant/child the burial takes place immediately with no special ceremony. For adults, the body is bathed. Sometimes the body may be clothed in white or traditional Chinese robes. Relatives and friends generally wish to see the body before the coffin is closed.

There is a minority who are accustomed to the traditional herbal remedies administered by Chinese physicians when they fall ill. Herbal medicine and acupuncture arc two common Chinese medical treatments.

Traditional Chinese medicine employs four diagnostic procedures as follows: first. looking at the patient's face, second, listening to the patient's voice, third, asking about the patient's dietary preferences, and fourth, feeling the patient's pulse. After evaluating the patient's complexion, emotional expression, pitch of voice, food consumed, and pulse rate, the herbal doctor then prescribes an appropriate list of herbs. Usually medical herbs are boiled in water for about two hours to make a bitter tea, which will be taken by the patient.

In general Chinese women have a comparatively shy and modest nature and, if possible, prefer to see a female doctor.

Diet

The Chinese diet is generally regarded as a healthy one. The Chinese are very concerned about eating habits which are seen as an important factor affecting health. There is a Chinese proverb *'Illness starts from what goes into one's mouth while trouble starts from what comes out of it.'* The majority of Chinese are not vegetarian.

There are several Chinese concepts of healthy eating habits. The most basic one is the balance of yin (feminine) and yang (masculine). Failure to maintain this balance is the root to many illnesses: excessive yin leads to weakness and excessive yang to restlessness manifested in inflammation and ulcers. Yin food includes fruits and vegetables whilst yang food includes meat. It is not uncommon to find that Chinese patients appear to lose their appetite during hospitalisation and may request food and rice to be brought into the hospital by their relatives and friends. This reflects their strong preference for home cooking.

DRUID/PAGAN

Roots

Paganism encompasses a diverse community with some groups concentrating on specific traditions, practices or elements such as ecology, witchcraft, Celtic traditions or certain gods. Wiccans, Druids, Shamans, Sacred Ecologists, Odinists and Heathens all make up parts of the Pagan community.

Druids are perhaps the most well known. They were ancient priests in a nature-based religion indigenous to Celtic Britain and other European regions. The actual term Druid means *'oak knowledge'*. Documented evidence (mostly from the Romans) of the activities of this group goes back to the third century BC. The Druids met annually and had great influence over political and social matters for their areas. They were well respected and revered members of their communities.

The actual term Druid refers to an elite class of respected Celtic officiates who were part of a powerful network which was based on common practice and outlook. It has been discovered that Druids performed the same tasks for their communities that a modern day scholar, judge, teacher or clergy member still performs today. The Druids also took part in divination and nature focused worship.

Druid orders meet up regularly and continue the traditions of reading Celtic poetry, while dressed in robes and wearing ancient Celtic symbols.   Held in exceptional honour are:

- The Bards are singers and poets, and the keepers of tradition.

- The Ovates are diviners and natural philosophers.

- The Druids are learned in natural and moral philosophy.

Beliefs

There is no definitive Druidic text. The Druidic culture was suppressed by ruling nations and lead to a necessity to keep the practices alive through myths, historical heroic stories and songs. Some of the basic beliefs of the modern-day Druid groups are:

- A belief in a multiplicity of gods and goddesses.

- The requirement of respect and love for nature

- A love for humanity and a belief that it is important to help fellow human beings.

- An importance is placed on celebrating the solar, lunar and other life cycles present in nature.

Festivals/Days of Observance

There are eight major Druidic festivals and observances; four correspond to the solar cycle and four to the lunar cycle. The festivals mark the seasonal equinoxes and traditional harvest/planting times. The most well know Druidic celebration takes place at Stonehenge during the summer solstice.

Sacred festivals associated with the livestock cycle, rather than the farming cycle, are:

- Samhuinn - between October 31st and November 2nd

- Imbolc - February 2nd

- Beltane - May 1st

- Lughnasadh - August 1st

Essential Information

Druids are believers in reincarnation. They believe that the soul is immortal and after a person dies, they are transported to the *'Otherworld'*. They also believe that that person will come back again in another human body. Members of the various Druid groups aim to dispose of their mortal remains in an environmentally-friendly and pollution-free way. Many will chose a natural burying ground.

While in hospital some Druids may wish to have a small white candle and simple holder or a small figure of a Goddess to hand.

Diet

Followers are expected to eat in the most ethically responsible way, respecting not only the environment but also honouring their own health and that of the community and descendants.

Roots

Hare Krishna is the popular name for the International Society of Krishna Consciousness (or ISKCON), a new religious movement based in Hinduism. His Divine Grace A. C. Bhaktivedanta Swami Prabhupada appeared in this world in 1896 in Calcutta, India. He first met his spiritual master, Srila Bhaktisiddhanta Sarasvati Gosvami, in Calcutta in 1922. Bhaktisiddhanta Sarasvati, a prominent religious scholar and the founder of sixty-four Gaudiya Mathas (Vedic institutes) in India, liked this educated young man and convinced him to dedicate his life to teaching Vedic knowledge. Srila Prabhupada became his student and, in 1933, his formally initiated disciple. ISKCON gained further publicity (and financial support) through the interest of the late Beatle, George Harrison.

Beliefs

The Hare Krishna worship the Hindu god Krishna, which means *'all attractive'*, as the one Supreme God. Their goal is *'Krishna consciousness'* and their central practice is the Hare Krishna mantra, thus the name. Hare Krishnas teach that we are living in an evil age, the age of Kali, but can attain salvation and a *'return to Godhead'* by means of permanent Krishna-consciousness. Chanting Hare Krishna is a way of seeking Krishna directly. The chant, called a mantra, is a vibration of sound that cleanses the mind, freeing it from anxiety and illusion. It is a mantra anyone can chant.

The most important sacred text for the Hare Krishna is the Hindu text Bhagavad Gita, the *'Song of the Lord,'* written around 250 BC. Beloved also by Gandhi and nearly all Hindus, the Gita tells the story of the warrior Arjuna and his encounter with Krishna.

Festivals/Days of Observance

Hare Krishnas are known for their public singing and dancing. Festivals are held in different venues throughout the year as are retreats. The biggest festival is Rathayatra, the International Society for Krishna Consciousness' biggest street festival - it features three huge, wooden chariots pulled by hand accompanied by singing, chanting, drums, cymbals, and dancing. It ends with a stage show, festival and delicious vegetarian prasadam (sanctified food offered to God). Major Hindu festivals are also observed (see page 4).

Essential Information

Members of the movement remain celibate except for purposes of procreation within marriage.

Male Hare Krishnas dress in white or saffron robes and shave their head except for a topknot; women wear brightly coloured saris.

It is deeply offensive to make fun of a devotee and part of the code clearly states this as well as a number of other offences against a devotee, for example:

- To kick or hit a devotee

- To criticise a devotee

- To anger or become angry at a devotee

- To envy a devotee

- To not be pleased to see a devotee

Members do not tolerate insensitivity because of caste. Congregational members of ISKCON put the movement's teachings about Krishna consciousness into practice while living a normal home and work life, and thus are likely to chant on the ward.

Diet

Followers who have devoted their lives to the movement and are *'temple based'* eat no meat, fish, or eggs nor drink alcohol or drugs (including caffeine) but other followers may also adhere to these strict principles.

HINDU

Roots

Hindu Religion originated in India about 4,000 years ago. There is a concept of the supreme spirit, Brahman, above the many divine manifestations. The three principal gods are:

- Brahma, who creates the universe.

- Vishnu, who preserves the universe

- Shiva, who destroys the universe.

Central to Hinduism are the beliefs in reincarnation and karma; the oldest scriptures are the Vedas. Bhaghavatd Gita, which is the essence of Vedas, is the Holy Book for Hindus. Uparishads are commentaries on Vedas. Temple worship is almost universally observed. There are over 805 million Hindus worldwide.

Beliefs/Scriptures

Brahma is the Creator. However, Brahma is not worshipped in the same way as other gods because it is believed that his work - that of creation - has been done. Hindus are often classified into three groups according to which form of Brahman they worship:

- Those who worship Vishnu (the preserver) and Vishnu's important incarnations Rama, Krishna and Narasimha.

- Those who worship Shiva (the destroyer). He is considered to be everything by those who worship him: creator, preserver and destroyer.

- The Veda collection of hymns and the epics were in existence before the Christian era. The Puranas, sacred historical texts dating from the 4th century AD, reflect the many cultural streams of India.

Hindu belief and ritual can vary greatly even between villages. Some deities achieve widespread popularity such as Krishna, Hanuman, Lakshmi, and Mahadevi; others, more localized and specialized, are referred to particularly in times of sickness or need. Hinduism includes teachings that condemn violence and war. The holy book Bhaghavad Gita advocates every human to do his duty.

Practice/Worship

Hindu worship, or puja, involves images (murtis), prayers (mantras) and diagrams of the universe (yantras).

Central to Hindu worship is the image, or icon, which can be worshipped either at home or in the temple. For ceremonial worship or puja, a Hindu needs flowers, fruits, leaves and sometimes coconuts. The majority of Hindu homes have a shrine where offerings are made and prayers are said. Some Hindus, but not all, wear the sacred thread (over the left shoulder and hanging to the right hip). This is cotton for the Brahmin (priest), hemp for the Kshatriya (ruler) and wool for the vaishya (merchants).

Hindu religious rites are classified into three categories:

- Nitya rituals are performed daily and consist in offerings made at the home shrine or performing puja to the family deities.

- Naimittika rituals are important but only occur at certain times during the year, such as celebrations of the festivals, thanksgiving and so on.

- Kamya are rituals which are optional but highly desirable.

Festivals/Days of Observance

- Ganesh Chaturthi: On this day Hindus all over the world will celebrate the birthday of Lord Ganesh (Ganesh Chaturthi) – the Elephant God.

- Hanuman Jayanti: This festival marks the birth of Hanuman, the Monkey God.

- Holi (the festival of colour/Spring festival): This is associated with Krishna lasting 2-5 days. Holi also celebrates creation and renewal.

- Rama Navami: Celebrates the birthday of the Lord Rama.

- Diwali: the Hindu festival of lights, is the most popular of all the festivals from South Asia, and is also the occasion for celebrations by Jains and Sikhs as well as Hindus. The main focus is Lakshmi, the Goddess of Wealth.

- Janamashtami: Celebrates the birthday of Lord Krishna, their most highly venerated God.

- Mahashivratri: Celebrates the birthday of the Lord Shiva.

- Makar Sakrani: first Hindu festival of the solar calendar year

- Navaratri/Durga Puja/Dassehra: One of the greatest Hindu festivals symbolising the triumph of good over evil. The festival takes place over nine nights of worship of the goddess Durga, the Hindus most important female deity.

- Raksha Bandhan is the Hindu festival that celebrates brotherhood and love. Hindu sisters tie a special thread called Rakti round their brother's wrists to protect them from evil.

- Rama Navami celebrates the birth of Lord Rama, son of King Dasharatha of Ayodhya.

- Vaisakhi - Common to all Hindus is that, at the time of Vaisakhi, people will go to the temple to pay their respect and seek blessings, and gifts and sweets will be exchanged between friends and family members.

- Varsha Pratipada is the Hindu Spring New Year

Essential Information

When considering abortion, the Hindu way is to choose the action that will do least harm to all involved: the mother and father, the foetus and society. There is no ban on birth control in Hinduism. There are several Hindu points of view on euthanasia and suicide. Most would say that assisting death brings bad karma because it violates the non violence principle but there are accepted Hindu ways to bring about death.

No religious law prohibits Hindus from donating their organs and tissues. Some Hindus practise the tradition of fasting during special occasions, such as holy days, new moon days and festivals.

Diet

Hinduism encourages being vegetarian and avoiding the eating of any animal meat or flesh. Some Hindus refrain from eating beef and pork, which are strictly prohibited in the Hindu diet code, but do eat other meats. A true devotee will refuse to accept any food that is not offered first to God. Once the food is offered to God, it is eaten as prasad or blessed food.

Before starting any daily meal, a devout Hindu first sprinkles water around the plate as an act of purification. Five morsels of food are placed on the side of the table to acknowledge the debt owed to the devta runa (divine forces) for their benign grace and protection.

For a child's birthday celebration, the sacred symbol 'OM' is added onto the birthday cake along with Happy Birthday. Also, a lamp is lit instead of having the child blow out the candles, symbolic of new life, a new beginning or the spreading of knowledge.

Tamasic food is leftover, stale, overripe, spoiled or other impure food, which is believed to produce negative emotions, such as anger, jealousy and greed.

Rajasic is food that is believed to produce strong emotional qualities, passions and restlessness in the mind. This category includes meat, eggs, fish, spices, onions, garlic, hot peppers, pickles and other pungent or spicy foods.

The most desirable type of food, Sattvic, is food that is non-irritating to the stomach and purifying to the mind; it includes fruits, nuts, whole grains and vegetables. These foods are believed to produce calmness and nobility, or what is known as an *'increase in one's magnetism.'*

ISLAMIC

Roots

The word Islam means submission, specifically to the will of God (Allah) which is a central element of faith. Its adherents are called Muslims. While there are several Muslim sects, all of them share the central belief that Prophet Muhammad is God's messenger, as were Abraham, Noah, Moses and Jesus before him, and that God's words are collected in the holy book, the Qur'an, as well as the previous reflections such as Psalms to David, Torah to Moses and Evangel to Jesus.

Beliefs

Islam is based on submission to the will of Allah, as revealed to the Prophet Mohammed through the Quran. Islamic belief stands on Five Pillars:

- Creed (belief in one God)

- Prayer

- Fasting/alms giving

- Pilgrimage

- Belief in the day of judgement

The prayer cycle begins at dawn and ends at dusk (times vary according to the season). After ritual washing, prayers are said five times a day facing Mecca (Makkah), reciting praises of God and supplicating in standing, bowing and prostrating positions. Shoes are removed and Muslims pray on a prayer mat or on clean ground. If possible, there should be a plain, private room for prayer. Young Muslims probably attend a Quranic school in the evenings and/or weekends to study the Quran and to receive instruction in the Islamic way of life. All prayers are said in Arabic.

Men over the age of 15 are expected to attend the mosque on a Friday; there are separate praying areas in the mosque for women.

The Sunni tradition (accepting the authority of Prophet Muhammed's first four caliphs – successors as head of the Muslim community) is the main group but some Muslims are Shia (the majority in Iran) which recognises only Prophet Mohammed's son-in-law, Ali (the fourth Caliph) as his rightful successor. followed by eleven others from Prophet Mohammed's progeny.

Festivals/Days of Observance

- Al-Hijra – Muslim New Year

- Ashura – Muslims commemorate the martyrdom of Prophet Muhammad's grandson, Hussain.

- Maulid al-Nabi – the celebration of the anniversary of the birth of the prophet Muhammad.

- Lailat-ul-Bara'h – The night of forgiveness. Muslims seek mutual forgiveness in preparation for Ramadan.

- Ramadan – during the month of Ramadan, Muslims fast from dawn to dusk and attend the mosque regularly. Fasting is seen as a way of increasing self-discipline. Children, women who are pregnant and people who are ill or disabled do not have to fast. Ramadan ends with the festival of Eid al Fitr.

- Eid al Fitr – this is the most important festival in the Muslim year (gifts of money or clothing are exchanged) and everyone celebrates.

- Eid al Adha – this feast of sacrifice is held in memory of the obedience shown by Abraham. Animals sacrificed for the feast provide food for the poor as well as being shared by friends and family.

Essential Information

When a child is born to Muslim parents, the first words it should hear are the call to prayer which should be whispered into its right ear by his or her father. Then the juice of a small piece of date or honey will be rubbed along its gums in accordance with the practice of the Prophet Muhammad. On the seventh day, a number of rituals are traditionally carried out: shaving the head, male circumcision, and the distribution of meat from a ceremonially slaughtered animal.

According to Islam, marriage is viewed as a social contract which binds couples together and obliges them to work to make each other happy. The actual ceremony is called a Nikah and it consists of readings from the Qur'an and the exchange of vows in front of witnesses. Marriages may vary widely in other respects. There is occasionally confusion on the issue of forced and arranged marriages. Arranged marriages are a cultural practice and some individual Muslims may find a partner in this way. A forced marriage is one performed without the consent of one or both of the parties, and they are not sanctioned by Islamic law, which states no action should be carried out under coercion.

Death is a time of sorrow but also of hopefulness, as Muslims believe death is not the end of a person's existence, just the end of life in this world. After death, prayers are said and the body is washed by a member of the family (same sex) and wrapped in a shroud. Prayers are said over the body, with the head facing to the right and it is buried facing Mecca - preferably within 24 hours. Muslims are never cremated. For the family, there is a three-day period spent at home, followed by mourning lasting about a month.

If possible a post-mortem should be avoided as this is not allowed under the Islamic code; if essential then the organs should be buried with the body.

If possible, a private place for prayer and a prayer mat should be provided with washing facilities. As well as ritual washing before prayers, Muslims require water to wash their private parts after every use of the toilet. Privacy is vital and many Muslims will not use a urinal. A Muslim will not normally answer when spoken to in the toilet, but will make a noise to indicate that s/he is still there. The left hand is used for washing after visiting the toilet, and the right hand for eating. Showers are often preferred to baths. After menstruation, women wash their whole bodies. Cleanliness is vital else a Muslim cannot perform the prayers if s/he is unclean.

Arrangements for worship at the mosque on a Friday, if leave allows this, should be made.

Diet

Muslims eat no pig products and will only eat other meat if it is slaughtered in accordance with Islamic law (Halal meat). Halal means lawful. Dairy products are allowed provided no non-Halal animal rennet has been used. Muslims will not eat food which has touched forbidden food. Haraam (or forbidden) foods also includes meat that has been sacrificed to idols, pork products, blood products, flesh without the blood drained from it, and from intoxicants. Seeds, nuts, vegetables and fruits are all halal. Alcohol is strictly forbidden.

Fasting, particularly during Ramadan, should be given consideration and help given with particular regard to the implications for medication.

JAINISM

Roots

Jainism is an ancient religion from India that teaches that the way to liberation and bliss is to live a life of harmlessness and renunciation. The aim of Jain life is to achieve liberation of the soul. Mahavira is regarded as the man who gave Jainism its present-day form. Lord Mahavir was the twenty-fourth and the last Tirthankara of the Jain religion. According to Jain philosophy, all Tirthankaras were born as human beings but they have attained a state of perfection or enlightenment through meditation and self realisation. They are the Gods of Jains. Tirthankaras are also known as Arihants or Jinas. Jainism has no priests. Its professional religious people are monks and nuns, who lead strict and ascetic lives.

Beliefs

Jains do not believe in a God or gods, but they do believe in divine beings who are worthy of worship.

The texts containing the teachings of Mahavira are called the Agamas. Jainism is a religion of self-help. The three guiding principles of Jainism (the three jewels) are right belief, right knowledge and right conduct. Jains believe that animals and plants, as well as human beings, contain living souls. Each of these souls is considered of equal value and should be treated with respect and compassion.

At the heart of right conduct for Jains lie the five great vows:

- Non-violence (Ahimsa) - not to cause harm to any living beings

- Truthfulness (Satya) - to speak the harmless truth only

- Non-stealing (Asteya) - not to take anything not properly given

- Chastity (Brahmacharya) - not to indulge in sensual pleasure

- Non-possession/Non-attachment (Aparigraha) - complete detachment from people, places, and material things.

Festivals/Days of Observance

Generally, festivals are celebrations and jubilations characterised by excitement, enthusiasm, enjoyments and entertainments; but the Jain festivals are characterised by renunciation, austerities, study of the scriptures, repetition of holy hymns, meditation and expressing devotion for the Paramatma.

- Paryushan Mahaparva & Das Lakshana - the real purpose of the Paryushan is to purify the soul, to look at our own faults, to ask for forgiveness for the mistakes and take vows to minimize our faults.

- The birthday of Mahavir - The birthday of Shraman Bhagwan, the last Tirthankar. On this occasion, a grand chariot procession, community worship, glorification of the Lord, discussions, discourses, seminars and devotional and spiritual activities are organised.

- Diwali - The whole of the night of Diwali should be spent in the recitation of holy hymns and in meditation on Shraman Bhagwan Mahavir. The Jains begin the new year with a glorification of Lord Gautam Swami; and listen with devotion to the nine Stotras holy hymns and with listening to the auspicious Rasa (epic poem) of Gautam Swami from their Guru Maharaj.

- Bhai Beej - The festival day for brothers.

- Jnan Panchami - The holy day for acquiring knowledge

- Ashadh Chaturdasi - During these months many austerities like renunciation, undertaking of religious ceremonies are organised with some rules in place concerning eating and drinking.

- Kartik Poornima - The full moon day of Kartik. Thousands of Jains go on pilgrimages on this day.

- Maun Ekadashi - The holy day for observing silence.

- Paush dashami - This day is famous as the birthday of Bhagwan Parshwanath. A grand fair takes place in Sankheswar which is a sacred place for Jains.

Essential Information

Jains believe in reincarnation and seek to attain ultimate liberation - which means escaping the continuous cycle of birth, death and rebirth so that the immortal soul lives forever in a state of bliss. The quality of a soul after death is determined by its karma at the time of death. Reincarnation if it is bad, and deliverance if it is good.

Santhara is the procedure in which a Jain stops eating with the intention of preparing for death. It is undertaken only when the inevitability of death is a matter of undisputed certainty.

Diet

Jains are strict vegetarians and live in a way that minimises their use of the world's resources.

JEHOVAH'S WITNESS

Roots

Jehovah's Witnesses had their modern-day start in the 1870s. At first, they were called Bible Students. But in 1931 they adopted the Scriptural name Jehovah's Witnesses (Isaiah 43:10). They are known for their door-to-door evangelistic work.

Beliefs

- The belief held by the Witnesses is that Jehovah is a holy God. In ancient times he was *'the Holy One of Israel,'* and as such he demanded that Israel be clean, unsullied. Jehovah laid down detailed laws so that the nation of Israel could identify and avoid wrongdoing. These laws included strict guidelines on morality. adultery and homosexual acts. Sex before marriage, adultery, bestiality, incest, and homosexuality are all serious sins.

Festivals/Days of Observance

Most congregations of Jehovah's Witnesses have meetings three times each week in a Kingdom Hall. These are usually simple structures built by Witness volunteers and there are no images or crucifixes.

In each congregation, there are elders, or overseers who take the lead in teaching in the congregation assisted by ministerial servants. Jehovah's Witnesses also hold large assemblies or conventions each year. At these times many congregations come together for a special programme of Bible instruction.

The most important religious event of the year for Jehovah's Witnesses is the commemoration of the Memorial of Christ's death, which takes place on the anniversary of the Last Supper, calculated according to the lunar calendar in use in Christ's time. They believe that this is the only observance commanded by Christ.

Witnesses do not celebrate Christmas or Easter because they believe that these festivals are based on (or massively contaminated by) pagan customs and religions. Witnesses do not celebrate birthdays or other secular festivals that originate in other religions. Witnesses should avoid forms of entertainment that could soil their minds. They also refuse military service, voting in elections. In countries with compulsory national service most Witnesses will accept civilian service as an alternative to military service. Certain civic obligations, such as jury service, are seen as a matter for individual decision according to the dictates of conscience.

Essential Information.

Baptism of new disciples is a regular part of each assembly or convention program and is not usually carried out until the age of 12. It is by complete immersion in the water.

Witnesses can only date and marry fellow believers of Christ. Witnesses do not approve of:

- masturbation

- sex outside marriage (includes petting and oral sex.)

- unchaperoned dates

- excessive public displays of affection

- homosexuality.

Jehovah's Witnesses believe the number of places available in heaven is restricted to 144,000. Apart from these chosen few, sometimes referred to as the *'little flock'* or *'great crowd'*, people and their souls cease to exist after death.

Jehovah requires that all witnesses abstain from blood. This means that they must not take into our bodies in any way at all other people's blood or even their own blood that has been stored. They will therefore not accept a blood transfusion. They will accept other kinds of medical treatment, such as transfusion of non blood products. They want to live, but they will not try to save their life by breaking God's laws.

A dying Witness patient may appreciate a visit from one of the Elders of their faith. They may be distressed or disappointed at the prospect of dying before Armageddon. Witnesses can choose to be buried or cremated.

Diet

For Jehovah's witnesses it is wrong to eat blood. It is also wrong for them to eat the meat of an animal that has not been properly bled. If an animal is strangled or dies in a trap, it should not be eaten. If it is speared or shot, it must be bled quickly if it is to be eaten.

JUDAISM

Roots

A Jew is the name given to members of the tribe of Judah, who were descendants of Abraham from about 2000 BC. Judaism is also a state that can be inherited; a child born to a Jewish mother, even if she never practises any of the things expected of a Jew, is considered to be Jewish. Recently, Liberal and Reform groups have extended this ruling to include children born to a Jewish father and non-Jewish mother; such children are considered to be Jewish by these groups, although not by Orthodox Jews.

Beliefs

The religious precepts of Judaism are simply to worship one God, to carry out the Ten Commandments, and to practise kindness and tolerance towards one's fellow human beings. The family has great importance in Jewish life.

Orthodox Jews believe that the Torah is the direct word of God and so it is perfect, divine, eternal and must be followed strictly.

Reform and Liberal/Progressive Jews believe that the Torah is the word of God translated by humans from an ancient culture and so, although the spirit of the law is eternal, the letter can – and often should – be tempered by modern circumstances. Reform and Progressive Jews may well observe the Sabbath, circumcise their male children and eat kosher food, but they are often otherwise fully integrated into whatever community they live in. They like to concentrate on what they believe is the heart of their religion, which is the relationship between the self and other Jews, between Jews and the rest of the world, and between the world and God.

The *'Scrolls of the Law'* are the Holy Books. At prayer some Orthodox men will wear the text of the Sherma strapped to their forehead and arm. A fringed shawl and small cap may be worn. Orthodox women may be particularly modest and may not wish others to look at their hair, or be observed by others in a teaching situation for example. There is an authorised Daily Prayer Book (Singers' Prayer Book).

Rabbis are considered to be the most prominent figures in any Jewish community. However, they are not elected leaders but are teachers, well versed in Jewish law (Halakah) and often act as a mediator in their community. They are the person that everyone goes to with their problems, the one who discusses and provides interpretation of Jewish law and who may carry out some ceremonies on behalf of their community.

Festivals/Days of Observance

Orthodox Jews are much stricter in their observance of Jewish law than liberal or reform Jews, especially between Friday evening and Saturday evening which is their Holy Day - The Sabbath. The main festivals/days of observance are:

- Days of Repentance - Days of Awe between Rosh Hashanah and Yom Kippur (10 days) when everyone gets a chance to repent.

- Hanukkah or Chanukah - the Jewish Festival of Lights.

- Passover - one of the most important religious festivals in the Jewish calendar, celebrated to commemorate the liberation of the Children of Israel who were led out of Egypt by Moses.

- Purim - commemorates the time when the Jewish people living in Persia were saved from extermination by the courage of a young Jewish woman called Esther.

- Rosh Hashanah - the Jewish New Year festival and commemorates the creation of the world.

- Shavuot - the time that the Jews received the Torah on Mount Sinai. It is considered a highly important historical event.

- Sukkot: - the years that the Jews spent in the desert on their way to the Promised Land.

- Tisha B'av - a solemn occasion because it commemorates a series of tragedies that have befallen the Jewish people over the years

- Tu B'Shevat (Tu Bishvat) - the Jewish *'New Year for Trees'*.

- Yom Hashoah is a day set aside for Jews to remember the Holocaust.

- Yom Kippur (The Day of Atonement) is the most sacred and solemn day of the Jewish year, and brings the Days of Repentance to a close.

Essential Information.

The treatment of male and female babies differs. Male babies go through a Brit Milah (circumcision) ceremony, where they are also publicly given their name. Female babies are usually named in the synagogue after a reading of the Torah.

Bar/Bat Mitzvah

Until they reach the age of adulthood (12 for girls, 13 for boys) Jewish children are not considered responsible for their actions. On reaching this age, the child automatically becomes bar mitzvah (son of the commandment) or bat mitzvah (daughter of the commandment). The occasion is often marked with a ceremony celebrating the child's coming of age. At the ceremony the child will normally make a speech, and there are festivities afterwards.

Marriage

The marriage ceremony is the culmination of a series of rituals that begin when the couple become engaged. These include announcing the union in the synagogue and ritual bathing. The ceremony takes place underneath a special canopy called a chupa.

Death

Jewish patients who are dying may wish to hear the 23rd Psalm recited – *The Lord is my Shepherd'*, and the special prayer, called The Sherma, which begins – *'Hear O Israel, The Lord is our God, The Lord is One'*. It may be comforting for them to hold the page on which the prayer is written. They may wish to pray with a Rabbi or make a silent confession.

After death the body should only be handled using disposable gloves, and touched as little as possible. The eyes should be closed and the jaw tied, keeping arms and hands straight at the sides. If practicable, this will be performed by one of the children of the deceased.

The body undergoes a purification process called Tahara, by which all dirt, fluids and marks are removed. It is then dressed and placed in a sealed coffin. After the burial, at which each of the mourners puts three shovelfuls of earth into the grave, a formal period of mourning begins. The mourners make a tear in their clothing to symbolise their broken heart and this clothing is worn for the following week-long period of Shiv'ah. During Shiv'ah, mourners do not shower or bathe, they remove jewellery and avoid wearing leather; men also stop shaving. A year after the death, the period of mourning is brought to a close and there is a ceremony marking the unveiling of the headstone.

It is considered to be one of the highest commandments for the community to tend the sick. It is generally poor taste to wish Jews a *'Merry/Happy Christmas.'* Although some Jews do celebrate Christmas as a secular event, Judaism discourages it and many Jews find Christmas greetings offensive. In keeping with the principle of the importance and holiness of the life of a person above all else, an abortion can be done in <u>all</u> cases if the woman's life is physically at risk. When in doubt a Rabbi should be consulted. Generally Orthodox and Chasidic women are more sensitive to needs of modesty and would like a woman doctor if possible

Diet

Orthodox Jews must eat only Kosher food and follow strict dietary laws: milk and meat must not be eaten together, meat must be killed according to Kosher ritual and must be from animals which chew the cud and have a cloven hoof, or from poultry. Pork, ham, bacon, or sausages, is forbidden, as are rabbit, fish without scales or fins and shellfish. If for any reason (perhaps in an emergency) a Kosher meal is not available, Jewish patients may prefer a vegetarian diet. Kosher means conforming to or prepared in accordance with Jewish dietary laws.

MORMON

Roots

The Church of the Latter Day Saints (Mormon) believes that Jesus Christ organised his church while on earth and died for the sins of the world. Through the Prophet Joseph Smith, the founder-leader, the angel Moroni lent him a set of gold plates from which he translated The Book of Mormon (1830). This tells of Jesus preaching in the United States after his resurrection. Smith was murdered in 1844, after which Brigham Young took over the leadership and led the *'saints'* to the Great Salt Lake in Utah. The last part of the Church's name, Latter-day Saints is used to distinguish the Saviour's Church today from the Christian Church in New Testament times. They see all human beings as children of the Father in heaven, regardless of their beliefs. Mormons operate the largest genealogical library in the world containing millions of volumes of birth, marriage, death, and other records.

Beliefs

Mormons use the authorised King James version of the Bible. Some of the basic principles and beliefs are:

- Charity - the pure love of Christ.

- Accountability - the ability of each person to choose right or wrong and to act freely.   Mormons believe this is a gift from God.

- Faith in Jesus Christ - regarded as one of the first principles and ordinances of the gospel of God.

- Fasting - a voluntary abstinence from food has been practised for centuries as a way for the Lord's people to humble themselves before Him and increase their ability to receive blessings.

- Forgiveness - an essential part of having happiness in this life and salvation in the life to come.

- Law of Chastity - a necessary set of commandments.

- Obedience - the first law of heaven.

- Prayer - the way by which any person can communicate directly with their Heavenly Father.

- Repentance (required for salvation) - the second principle of the Gospel in Mormon doctrine.

- Sacrament - a ceremony of eating bread and drinking water which are symbols, or reminders, of the body and blood of Christ.

- Tithing, or tithe, means a tenth part - the paying of tithes to the Lord and his church.

- Important truths regarding the ce*ntrality of the family and its* eternal destiny.

Festivals/Days of Observance

The Sabbath Day is Sunday in the Mormon Church. Most Mormon families will spend a substantial part of Sunday in meetings and worship with their community. Monday is often reserved for Family Home Evening. Mormons really only celebrate two religious festivals: Easter and Christmas. An additional festival is Pioneer Day, on 24 July. This celebrates the arrival of the first Latter-day Saint pioneers in the Salt Lake Valley in 1847. Church members fast each month (on the first Sunday) by going without food and drink for two consecutive meals.

Essential Information

Baptism is very important in Mormonism.

Joseph Smith, the founder of the Mormon church, said the idea of *'plural marriage'* was revealed to him by God. Among early Mormon pioneers, 20-25% of families were polygamous. LDS president Wilford Woodruff announced an official end to the practice of polygamy in 1890. The Church of Jesus Christ of Latter-day Saints believes that a dead person can be baptised by proxy, which means that a Mormon can be baptised on behalf of someone who has already died. Except where it isn't allowed, Mormons prefer to bury their dead rather than cremate them.

Mormons believe their bodies are sacred gifts from God which are made after the likeness of the Lord and should be treated as sacred. Members of the Mormon Church are taught from a young age to respect their bodies as temples wherein the Spirit of the Lord can reside.

Diet

Latter-day Saints caution their members against using tobacco, consuming alcohol, tea and coffee. They interpret the misuse of drugs (illegal, legal, prescription or controlled) as a violation of the health code known as the *'Word of Wisdom.'* Tobacco or alcohol users cannot hold most Church offices or attend special non-Sabbath day services in Latter-day Saints' temples. The dietary aspects of their Word of Wisdom are left up to individuals.

ORTHODOX CHRISTIAN

Roots

The word Orthodox means the correct belief or right thinking. It takes the meaning from the Greek vocabulary: Orthos meaning *right* and the word doxa meaning *belief*. The Orthodox Church shares much with the other Christian churches in the belief that God revealed himself in Jesus Christ, and a belief in the incarnation of Christ, his crucifixion and resurrection. The Orthodox Church differs substantially in the way of life doctrine and worship. The two most widely known Orthodox traditions are the Greek and Russian.

Although initially the Eastern and Western Christians shared the same faith, the two traditions began to divide after the seventh Ecumenical Council in 787 AD and is commonly believed to have finally split over the conflict with Rome in the so called Great Schism in 1054.

Beliefs

A prominent place is always assigned to Holy Icons, placed in prominent places throughout the church building. The walls and ceiling are covered with iconic murals. The Orthodox faithful prostrate themselves before Icons, kiss them, and burn candles before them.

The Bible of the Orthodox Church is the same as that of most Western Churches, except that its Old Testament is based not on the Hebrew, but on the ancient Jewish translation into Greek called the Septuagint. Eastern Christianity stresses a way of life and belief that is expressed particularly through worship. Monasticism is a central part of the Orthodox faith.

Festivals/Days of Observance

At the centre of worship and belief is the Eucharist surrounded by the Divine Offices or the Cycle of Prayer. These prayers are sung particularly at sunset and dawn and at certain other times during the day and night.

Personal prayer plays an important part in the life of an Orthodox Christian.

There are four main fasting periods:

- The Great Fast or the period of Lent

- The Fast of the Apostles: Eight days after Pentecost until 28th June. The ends with the Feast of Saint Peter and Saint Paul.

- The Dormition Fast which begins on 1st August and ends on the 14th August

- All over the world, throughout the month of January, Orthodox Christians will assemble to bless the waters. Sometimes they simply bless a large tub of water in church or go in procession to a spring, stream, lake or even to the sea.

- All Wednesdays and Fridays are expected to be days of fasting.

Essential Information

The Orthodox Church practises baptism by full immersion.

Marriage in the Orthodox Church is forever. In the Orthodox marriage rite, the bride and groom offer their lives to Christ and to each other - literally as crowned martyrs. The Orthodox Christian faith holds to the biblical teaching that sexual intercourse is reserved for marriage.

After appropriate pastoral counsel, divorce may be allowed when avenues for reconciliation have been exhausted. If there is a remarriage, the service for a second marriage includes prayers offering repentance for the earlier divorce, asking God's forgiveness, and protection for the new union.

Funeral planning is important as it enables family and friends to come together to express feelings of love, grief and sadness and helps family and friends accept the reality of death. For the Orthodox Christian there is no choice as according to the Holy Canons of the Church, the body of a deceased Christian must be returned to the earth. Cremation is specifically forbidden.

QUAKER

Roots

The Religious Society of Friends, (otherwise known as Quakers), was founded by George Fox (1624 - 1691). Friends observe no sacraments and have no dogmas or creeds. They believe, simply, that there is something of God in everyone, and that in the stillness of the corporate Meeting for Worship they can meet God's real presence and know something of his Will.

Beliefs

Attitudes to spoken prayer and to the Bible vary widely; some Friends are clearly *'Christ focused'* in their beliefs, while others are not.

Quakers are especially active in peace work, human rights and social reform and have a long-standing historic involvement with the criminal justice system on both sides of the bars.

Quakers' attitude is always non-violent and challenges war, violence and injustice by focusing on the root causes of oppressive use of power, fear and separation. This commitment to non violence is known as *'Quaker peace testimony'*.

The Friends consider that the values of trust, autonomy, consent and truth need to underpin mental health legislation and that everyone has the potential for psychological growth and development through loving relationships. No one is born evil.

Quakers recognise the equal worth and unique nature of every person.

Essential Information

Silent worship is the common experience, and the offer of a shared silence with an ill friend will usually be welcomed. Equally, Friends would normally wish to have a Meeting for Worship in the event of a stillbirth. the offer of a shared silence with bereaved relatives would be appropriate.

Quakers do not baptise or practise Eucharistic communion.

Friends have no priesthood. The Overseers are charged with pastoral oversight of the members of the Meeting, and work closely with any hospital in relation to a Friend in hospital.

Diet

Because of the absence of dogma, there are no preferences of diet, clothing or occupation that would be seen as distinctively Quaker. However, many Friends seek to live as simply as possible, and a growing number would be vegetarian. Quakers typically avoid drinking, drugs, smoking, and oath-taking (swearing).

RASTAFARIAN

Roots

Rastafarianism is a relatively recent development and is of African origin. However, the movement started in Jamaica and is thought to have been inspired by the philosophy of Marcus Garvie. He advocated pride in the black consciousness and the resistance to worldwide white domination. Garvey reportedly said *'Look to Africa for the crowning of a black king. He will be the redeemer.'* When Haile Selassie was crowned King of Kings, Lord of Lords, Conquering Lion of the Tribe of Judah, Garvey's followers took this to be sign that the scriptures were about to be fulfilled. His Imperial Majesty Haile Selassi I (also known as Rastafari) was treated as the black messiah of whom Garvey had spoken.

Beliefs

Through the way they dress, their dreadlocks, their music and language, Rastafarians assert their right to define themselves. They determine how they should live, who they are and the values they should follow. There is therefore no defined system of beliefs.

Rastafarians are deeply religious people who spend a great deal of time reading and analysing the Bible in search of truth. Great emphasis is placed on the love of God and the love of one's neighbour.

Festivals/Days of Observance

- January 6/7 - Christmas

- July 23 - Haile Selassie's birthday

- Ethiopian New Year's Day (September)

- Nov 2 - Coronation of Haile Selassie

Essential Information

When a child is born into the Rastafari tradition he or she is blessed by elders in the community, during a Nyabingi session of drumming, chanting and prayer.

In Rastafari there is no formal marriage structure. A Rastafari man and woman who live together are regarded as husband and wife (unless, of course, they are related in some other way, such as mother and son). If marriage does take place it is regarded as a social occasion rather than a religious event.

In Rastafari there is no funeral ceremony to mark the end of life. Rastafarians believe that reincarnation follows death, and that life is eternal.

Diet

By nature Rastafarians are vegetarian. Many will find hospital food a source of contention as they wish to eat natural, organic food. If possible and practical, an agreement may be reached with a friend or relative to bring in food.

Rastafarians see meat, especially pork (swine) as being harmful to man. Shellfish, scale less fish and snails are not allowed, nor are products of the vine (wine, raisins, currants or grapes). Canned foods and preservatives are also avoided as they are considered to be polluted; frozen food is however acceptable

Some Rastafarians are deeply against coming into hospital and follow the example of Bob Marley who, although suffering from cancer of the toe, did not go to hospital as he believed this was God's will.

Rasta language is based on Jamaican patois and creates greater cohesion and solidarity among the members while defining the boundary between Rastas and non-Rastas.

The smoking of Ganja (marijuana) has great religious significance to some Rastafarians and is thought to be a source of revelation, inspiration, nutrition, relaxation and healing. The growing of dreadlocks also has great religious significance and is in accordance with the laws of nature.

One of the more obvious symbols of the Rastafarians are colours. These are red, gold, and green. The colour red stands for the Church Triumphant which is the church of the Rastas. It also symbolises the blood that martyrs have shed in the history of the Rastas. The gold represents the wealth of the homeland. Green represents the beauty and vegetation of Ethiopia, the promised land. Sometimes black is used to represent the colour of Africans, from whom 98% of Jamaicans are descended.

The traditional music of the Rastafarian religion is Nyabingi, consisting of chanting and drumming. Rastafari was popularised by reggae artists, including Bob Marley.

SHINTO

Roots

Shinto is an ancient Japanese religion. Starting about 500 BC (or earlier) it was originally *"an amorphous mix of nature worship, fertility cults, divination techniques, hero worship and shamanism."* Its name was derived from the Chinese words "shin tao" ("The Way of the Gods") in the 8th Century Unlike most other religions, Shinto has no real founder, no written scriptures, no body of religious law, and only a very loosely-organised priesthood.

Beliefs

Shinto creation stories tell of the history and lives of the *"Kami"* (deities). Among them was a divine couple, Izanagi-no-mikoto and Izanami-no-mikoto, who gave birth to the Japanese islands. Their children became the deities of the various Japanese clans. Amaterasu Omikami (Sun Goddess) was one of their daughters. She is the ancestress of the Imperial Family and is regarded as the chief deity. Her shrine is at Ise. Her descendants unified the country. Her brother, Susano, came down from heaven and roamed throughout the earth. He is famous for killing a great evil serpent.

Shinto does not have its own moral code. Shintoists generally follow the code of Confucianism.

- Ancestors are deeply revered and worshipped.

- All of humanity is regarded as *"Kami's child."* Thus all human life and human nature is sacred.

- Believers revere *"musuhi"*, the Kamis' creative and harmonising powers. They aspire to have *"makoto"*, sincerity or true heart. This is regarded as the way or will of Kami.

- Morality is based upon that which is of benefit to the group. *"Shinto emphasizes right practice, sensibility, and attitude."*

There are "Four Affirmations" in Shinto:

- Tradition and the family - The family is seen as the main mechanism by which traditions are preserved. Their main celebrations relate to birth and marriage.

- Love of nature - Nature is sacred; to be in contact with nature is to be close to the Gods. Natural objects are worshipped as sacred spirits.

- Physical cleanliness - Followers of Shinto take baths, wash their hands, and rinse out their mouth often.

- "Matsuri" - The worship and honour given to the Kami and ancestral spirits.

Essential Information

The standardised Shinto wedding ritual is very recent. Death is seen as impure and conflicting with the essential purity of Shinto shrines. Shinto worship can take place in the home or in shrines. Ritual is very important.

- Harae *(purification rites)-* Purity can be restored through specific Shinto rituals and personal practices that cleanse both body and mind.

- Hatsumiyamairi - This marks the first shrine visit.

- Shichigosan - This is an occasion for giving thanks for children of the ages three, five and seven.

- Seijin Shiki - A celebration for new adults upon reaching 20 years old.

SIKH

Roots

The Sikh religion was founded by Guru Nanak in the Punjab, India, in the 15th century. Guru Nanak was followed by a further nine gurus. The life story of Guru Nanak and the early Gurus are contained in the Janam-Sakhis (life stories) written 50 years after Guru Nanak's death.

Beliefs

Sikhs believe that the eternal Guru took material form in Guru Nanak and, after his death, was embodied in the second Guru, Guru Angad Nev, and then in each of the successive Gurus. The last of these, Guru Gobind Singh, established the Khalsa (pure) order of Sikhs.

The most important thing in Sikhism is the internal religious state of the individual. It is a monotheistic religion (belief in only one God, who is without form or gender) which stresses the importance of doing good actions rather than merely carrying out rituals, which in themselves have no value. Everyone has direct access to God and everyone is equal before God. Sikhs can pray at anytime and anywhere, but there are set prayers to be performed in the morning, evening and before going to sleep. Sunday is the main day for worship in the Gurdwara.

Sikhs believe that the way to lead a good life is to:

- Keep God in heart and mind at all times

- Live honestly and work hard and care for others

- Treat everyone equally

- Be generous to the less fortunate

- Serve others

Festivals/Days of Observance

The main Sikh festivals/holy days are:

- Diwali is particularly important to Sikhs as it celebrates the release from prison of the sixth guru, Hargobind Singh in 1619

- Gurpurbs are festivals that are associated with the lives of the Gurus. The birthday of Guru Gobind Singh, the tenth and last Guru of the Sikhs and founder of the Khalsa (the brotherhood of the Sikhs) is celebrated (February).

- On Hola Mohalla, Sikhs practise military exercises and hold mock battles

- Vaisakhi, also spelled Baisakhi, is one of the most important dates in the Sikh calendar. It is the Sikh New Year festival and is celebrated on April 13 or 14.

- In October Sikhs honour the Guru Granth Sahib as a living Guru.

Essential Information

The birth of a child is not marked with any specific religious ceremony, but the infant is usually taken to the Gurdwara for prayers and a blessing. A child's name is traditionally chosen at the Gurdwara by opening the Guru Granth Sahib at random and reciting the first paragraph on the opened page. The family chooses a name starting with the first letter of the first word, and announces it to the whole congregation.

The Amrit ceremony marks a Sikh's induction into the Khalsa order. During the ceremony there are prayers, hymns and readings. The candidate for initiation commits to a set of rules of behaviour and drinks amrit (a mix of sugar and water stirred with a double edged sword), which is also sprinkled on their hair and eyes. After this ceremony the initiate wears the physical symbols of Khalsa at all times and abides by the Khalsa code of conduct.

The five physical articles of faith (the five Ks) are visible manifestations of a Sikh's induction into the Khalsa path. They are:

- Kesh - uncut bodily hair

- Kangha - a comb

- Kara - a steel bracelet

- Kachha - special underwear

- Kirpan - a ceremonial sword

Parents and relatives still play a key role in arranging the marriage although many young people now have a greater say in the choice of a partner. The Sikh marriage ceremony, known as Anand Karaj, usually takes place in the morning and is conducted by an Amritdhari Sikh (one who has been initiated into the Khalsa). The couple are reminded of their obligations to each other and vow mutual fidelity in the presence of the Guru Granth Sahib. A Sikh marriage is an insoluble sacrament so divorce is rare.

After death, the body is washed, traditionally by the family, and then taken to the Gurdwara before it is cremated. The family then undertake a continuous reading of the Guru Granth Sahib either at the family home or in the Gurdwara. These rites last about a week, after which the mourners come together and share blessed food. Many choose to scatter the ashes in India. The body of a still born child or late miscarriage should be given to the parents so that they may have a traditional funeral. Both widows and widowers may remarry.

Sikh women (especially the older generation) prefer to be treated for gynaecological conditions by a female doctor. Consideration should also be given to their modesty when, for example, the patient is being prepared for X-ray, surgery, medical examination or washing/bathing Requests to a man to remove his turban or underwear in public should be made with discretion.

Sikhs are accustomed to washing after visiting the toilet so, if using a bedpan, they should be given a bowl of water to wash in.

Diet

The majority of Sikhs are vegetarian, although dietary requirements are the choice of the individual. For all Sikhs, the consumption of meat from cows is prohibited, as is eating the flesh of any animal killed according to the Halal method. Sikhs who are initiated into the Khalsa abstain from stimulants and drugs, and are prohibited from eating eggs, meat and fish. Alcohol is also forbidden.

TAOISM

Roots

Tao (pronounced 'Dow') can be roughly translated into English as *path*, or *the way*. The founder of Taoism is believed by many to be Lao-Tse (604-531 BCE), a contemporary of Confucius.

Beliefs

Because Taoism is a polytheistic religion there is not one single god to worship or honour. Religious adherents often choose one of many gods that is especially useful at a particular time. Each of these deities represents different qualities. Principles are:

- The One is the essence of Tao, the essential energy of life, the possession of which enables things and beings to be truly themselves and in accord with the Tao.

- Wu and Yu are non-being and being, or not-having and having. Wu also implies inexhaustibility or limitlessness.

- Te is usually translated as virtue.

- Tzu Jan is usually translated naturalness or spontaneity.

- Wu Wei means living by or going along with the true nature of the world - or at least without obstructing the Tao - letting things take their natural course. Taoists live lives of balance and harmony.

- Tao Te Ching does not stop a person living a proactive life but their activities should fit into the natural pattern of the universe, and therefore need to be completely detached and disinterested and not ego-driven.

- Yin Yang is the principle of natural and complementary forces, patterns and things that depend on one another and do not make sense on their own. These may be masculine and feminine, but they could be darkness and light (which is closer to the original meaning of the dark and light sides of a hill), wet and dry or action and inaction. The yin yang concept is not the same as Western dualism, because the two opposites are not at war, but in harmony.

Festivals/Days of Observance

At the heart of Taoist ritual is the concept of bringing order and harmony to many layers of the cosmos: the cosmos as a whole (the world of nature). Taoist rituals involve purification, meditation and offerings to deities. The details of Taoist rituals are often highly complex and technical and therefore left to the priests, with the congregation playing little part. The rituals involve the priest (and assistants) in chanting and playing instruments (particularly wind and percussion), and also dancing. One major Taoist ritual is the *chiao* (*jiao*), a rite of cosmic renewal, which is itself made up of several rituals. Reciting passages from the Tao Te Ching has been a spiritual practice for over 2000 years.

Diet

Taoism recommends a healthy natural diet without chemicals and additives. Plenty of whole grain foods, fresh locally grown vegetables, beans, nuts, seeds, soya bean curd (tofu), soya, rice and soya milk and soya yoghurt, fresh fruit and honey. Soy Sauce is also popular.

ZOROASTRIAN

Roots

The religion was founded by Zarathushtra (Zoroaster in Greek; Zarthosht in India and Persia). Historians and religious scholars generally date his life sometime between 1500 and 1000 BCE. He lived in Persia, modern day Iran. One has to be born into the religion.

Beliefs

The motto of the faith is *'good thoughts, good words, good deeds.'* The Zorastrian holy book is called the Avesta. This includes the original words of their founder Zarathushtra, preserved in a series of five hymns, called the Gathas. The Gathas are abstract sacred poetry, directed towards the worship of the One God, understanding of righteousness and cosmic order, promotion of social justice and individual choice between good and evil. Their worship includes prayers and symbolic ceremonies.

Zoroastrian rituals are conducted before a sacred fire. Adherents regard fire as a symbol of their God, and they cherish the light that it produces. Light is seen as energy, a natural force that is powerful and necessary for survival. Zoroastrians traditionally pray several times a day. Some wear a kusti, which is a cord knotted three times, to remind them of the maxim, *'Good Words, Good Thoughts, Good Deeds'*.

Festivals/Days of Observance

Zoroastrians have seven obligatory feasts, six of which are the gahanbars. Noruz is the Iranian New Year, which is celebrated each year at the Spring Equinox, around March 21. It is the most important holiday in the Zoroastrian calendar, and brings with it a wealth of symbolism, history, myth, and joyous festivities. There are many layers of meaning to Noruz: astronomical, mythical, historical, ritual, and spiritual. Purification is strongly emphasized in Zoroastrian rituals. Zoroastrians focus on keeping their minds, bodies and environments pure in the quest to defeat evil (Angra Mainyu).

Festivals/Days of Observance

- Jamshedi Noruz – New Year's Day according to the Fasli calendar used in Iran.

- Zartusht-no-Diso (May) – the commemoration of the death of the Prophet Zarathustra.

- No Ruz (August) – New Year's Day on the Shenshai calendar

- Khordad Sal (August) – commemoration of the birthday of Zarathustra.

Essential Information

The Navjote is the initiation ceremony where a child between the ages of seven and twelve receives his or her sudreh (a long, clean, white cotton shirt.) and kusti (a cord knotted three times) which is wrapped around the outside of the sudreh.

There are two stages to a Zoroastrian wedding. Marriage is considered to be an event which must be celebrated n the presence of an assembly (Anjoman), which can bear witness to the event.

Zoroastrianism does not teach or believe in reincarnation or karma. Zoroastrians believe that after life on earth, the human soul is judged by God as to whether it did more good or evil in its life. Those who chose good over evil go to what Zarathushtra referred to simply as the *'best existence'* or heaven, and those who chose evil go to the *'worst existence'* or hell. At the end of time everything and everyone will be purified, even the souls in hell - so hell is not eternal.

Diet

Many Zoroastrians follow a semi-vegetarian diet without beef, pork and poultry.

Language	Where Spoken (Major)
Arabic	Middle East, Arabia, North Africa
Bengali	Bangladesh, Eastern India
Burmese	Myanmar
Cantonese	Southern China
English	USA, UK, Australia, Canada, New Zealand
Farsi (Persian)	Iran, Afghanistan, Central Asia
French	France, Canada, West Africa, Central Africa
German	Germany, Austria, Central Europe
Gujarati	Western India, Kenya
Hindi	North and Central India
Italian	Italy, Central Europe
Japanese	Japan
Javanese	Indonesia
Kannada	Southern India
Kutchi	India (state of Gujarat)
Korean	Korean Peninsula
Malay, Indonesian	Indonesia, Malaysia, Singapore
Mandarin	China, Malaysia, Taiwan
Marathi	Western India
Polish	Poland, Central Europe
Portuguese	Brazil, Portugal, Southern Africa
Punjabi	Pakistan, India
Russian	Russia, Central Asia
Spanish	The Americas, Spain
Tamil	Southern India, Sri Lanka, Malaysia
Telugu	Southern India
Thai	Thailand, Laos
Turkish	Turkey, Central Asia
Urdu	Pakistan, India
Vietnamese	Vietnam, China
Wu	China

Languages	Hindi	Urdu	Punjabi	Gujarati	Bengali	Kutchi
Hindi		Almost All	Quite a lot	A little	Nothing	A little
Urdu	Almost all		Quite a lot	A little	Nothing	A little
Punjabi	A little	Quite a lot		A little	Nothing	A little
Gujarati	Quite a lot	A little	A little		Nothing	Quite a lot
Bengali	A little	A little	Nothing	Nothing		Nothing
Kutchi	A little	A little	A little	Quite a lot	Nothing	

Fear of getting it wrong or offending can cause confusion as to what are acceptable terms to use. It has to be remembered that terms are evolving and developing all the time. What is in common use at a particular time may be seen to be unacceptable in the future. These terms are not prescriptive.

- Anti-discrimination - Refers to an approach that is taken which challenges unfair treatment of individuals or groups based on a specific characteristic of that group, e.g. colour, age, disability etc.

- Anti-racist - A general term describing an activity, event, policy or organisation combating racism in any form.

- Black - This is a term that has undergone considerable change and development. As several different meanings are currently in use, it should be used with caution and understanding. Additionally, there has also been a desire from visible minority ethnic peoples to self-define themselves, including being defined as members of groups distinguished by ethnicity, nationality or religion. In recent years 'black' has been used less often in this all-encompassing sense, being replaced by such terms as 'black and Asian', 'black and ethnic minority', 'black/minority ethnic'. The term is still used in its broad ideological, inclusive sense but is increasingly used to refer to people of African and Caribbean origin. Currently classifications are confused, with some ethnic groups being categorised under 'colour' as in 'Black African/Black Caribbean' and other ethnic groups such as Asians being categorised not under colour codes but according to national origins such as 'Indian/Bangladeshi/Pakistani'.

- Black minority ethnic (BME) - A term used to describe people from minority groups, particularly those who are viewed as having suffered racism or are in the minority because of their skin colour and/or ethnicity. This term has evolved over time becoming more common as the term 'black' has become less all-inclusive of those experiencing racial discrimination.

- Coloured - This usage is now outdated, though it is a term that is still fairly commonly employed. The term tends to suggest that, in the user's view, 'colour' is an attribute possessed by all skin types other than white and can therefore be used as an identifier for 'non-white' people. Today such usage tends to cause offence, or, at best, to indicate a naive or patronising approach in a multi-ethnic environment. A common term used in North America to denote all non-white people is 'people of colour'. This term is not perceived as derogatory and aims to be inclusive of non-white people as well as people of mixed parentage and ancestry.

- Culture - The total range of social values, beliefs and behaviours of an identifiable group of people with a shared background and traditions which influence and characterise members of that group's or society's core outlooks and activities. Culture is often closely linked to race and ethnicity.

- Discrimination - Racial discrimination is the treating of a particular group of people, or individuals belonging to that group, less favourably than others on grounds of their supposed race, colour, nationality, or ethnic or national origins. In Britain, the Race Relations Act (1976) and its Amendment (2000) make both direct and indirect discrimination illegal.

- Diversity - A variety of something such as opinion, colour, or style. When used to promote social inclusiveness, this term is often used to mean diversity within society of colour, culture, gender, sexual orientation, ability, socio-economic status, type of area (urban/rural), age, faith and/or beliefs.

- Equality - The state of being equal.

- Equal opportunities - A descriptive term for an approach intended to give equal access to an environment or benefits or equal treatment for all.

- Ethnic/Ethnicity - 'Ethnic' means 'relating to or characteristic of a human group having certain key features in common'. It is derived from the Greek 'ethnos' meaning a (non-Greek) 'race'.

- Ethnic minority - The term 'ethnic minority' is mainly used to denote people who are in the minority within a defined population on the grounds of 'race', colour, culture, language or nationality. I

- Inclusion - The act of including or the state of being included. This has to go beyond physical inclusion to inclusion at social, cultural and institutional levels.

- Positive discrimination - This term refers to a process which seeks to redress the under-representation of defined 'racial' groups in particular occupations, status groups (for example, managers) and courses by skewing competition for scarce opportunities in favour of minority ethnic candidates, providing they possess the required qualifications. on those at the lower end of the social scale, and in various states affirmative action measures were repealed in the 1990s.

- Race - This is a controversial term, which comes from historical attempts to categorise people according to their skin colour and physical characteristics. The word has no scientific basis for divisions into biologically determined groups. Individuals, not 'races', are the main sources of human variation. It is, however, in everyday use and is enshrined in legislation in the Race Relations Acts. The word 'race' is used with quotation marks by some authors as an acknowledgement that it is a controversial and contested term.

- Racism - Broadly used to refer to the ideology of superiority of a particular race over another. This notion of superiority is then applied to and embedded in structures, practices, attitudes, beliefs and processes of a social grouping which then serve to further perpetuate and transmit this ideology. Racism appears in several, often interrelated, forms, e.g. personal, cultural, and institutional.

- Xenophobia - An irrational fear or hatred of foreigners or strangers or of their politics or culture.

www.ingramcontent.com/pod-product-compliance
Lightning Source LLC
Chambersburg PA
CBHW050354180526

45159CB00005B/2013